Lean and Green Recipes

TASTY AND HEALTHY RECIPES TO LOSE WEIGHT EASILY BY USING A SIMPLE LEAN AND GREEN COOKBOOK.

Patricia Parker

professional before attempting any techniques outlined in this book.

By reading this document, the reader agrees that under no circumstances is the author responsible for any losses, direct or indirect, which are incurred as a result of the use of information contained within this document, including, but not limited to, — errors, omissions, or inaccuracies.

TABLE OF CONTENT

Introduction

The lean and green diet is a healthy eating pattern that helps you lose weight and maintain health. You will consume a combination of purchased and homemade "lean and green" meals and processed foods, called "supplies". With this diet, there is no need to count calories or carbohydrates.

This diet was designed not only to help you lose weight but also to improve lipid and blood sugar levels, as well as better overall health.

The Lean and Green diet subscribes to the idea that eating several small meals or snacks every day leads to manageable and sustained weight loss, and ultimately habit change. The thinking is that instead of eating three huge meals every day, you'll never get that hungry because you're eating six or seven small, filling, and nutritious meals throughout the day. While this may work well for some people, we're all different and there isn't a ton of convincing research to back this method up. The efficacy of eating small meals and found that, ultimately, weight loss is directly related to restricting calories, and the timing and sizing of the meals themselves don't have a meaningful impact on weight loss.

When it comes to successful long-term weight loss, experts seem to agree on one thing: The emotional and behavioral aspects of eating not just the specific meals you're eating are incredibly important. They also stress the importance of looking at whole-body wellness as a path to safe and sustainable weight loss.

What To Eat

- Lean and Green fuelings
- Lean meats
- Greens and other non-starchy vegetables
- Healthy fats
- Low-fat dairy, fresh fruit, and whole grains

What Not To Eat

- Indulgent desserts
- High-calorie additions
- Sugary beverages
- Alcohol

What Kinds Of Foods Can I Eat On the Lean and Green Diet?

- Lean meats, like turkey, lamb, or chicken
- Fish and shellfish, like salmon, crab, shrimp
- Tofu

- Low-carb veggies, including spinach, cauliflower, mushrooms, and cabbage
- Healthy fats, like avocados and pistachios
- Sugar-free beverages and snacks, including coffee and tea
- Vegetable oils
- Eggs

What Foods Should I Avoid On the Lean and Green Diet?

- Fried foods
- Refined grains, like white bread, pasta, and white
- rice Alcohol
- Butter
- Coconut oil
- Milk
- Cheese

RECIPES

Cauliflower Casserole

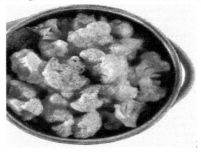

Prep Time: 30 mins **Cook Time:** 30 mins **Total Time:** 1 hr

MAKES 6 SERVINGS

INGREDIENTS

- ➤ 8 slices of bacon, fried crispy
- ➤ 1 large head cauliflower, cut into florets
- ➤ 1/2 cup sour cream
- ➤ 1/2 cup mayonnaise
- ➤ 1 tablespoon ranch seasoning
- ➤ ¼ teaspoon black pepper
- ➤ 1 cup shredded Colby & Monterey jack cheese
- ➤ 1 cup sharp cheddar cheese
- ➤ 6 tablespoons chopped fresh chives, divided

INSTRUCTIONS

1. Preheat oven to 370 degrees.
2. Spray an 11×7 baking dish with non-stick cooking spray.

3. Fry bacon in a large skillet until crispy and crumble. Set aside.

4. Steam cauliflower until tender, about 15 to 20 minutes.

5. Combine your sour cream, mayonnaise, ranch seasoning, black pepper in a large bowl.

6. Add the steamed cauliflower florets, 1/2 of the bacon, 1 cup sharp cheddar cheese, and 3 tablespoons chives; mix well.

7. Transfer mixture to the prepared baking dish and top with your Colby & Monterey jack cheese and the other half of the bacon.

8. Cover the dish with foil and bake for 20 minutes. Remove foil and bake another 5-10 minutes or just until cheese is bubbly and beginning to brown.

9. Garnish casserole with remaining chives.

Bok Choy with Soy Sauce

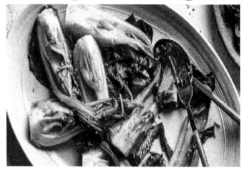

Prep Time: 10 mins **Cook Time:** 8 mins **Total Time:** 18 mins

MAKES 4 SERVINGS

INGREDIENTS

- ➢ 1 pound baby bok choy
- ➢ 2 tablespoon soy sauce
- ➢ 2 tablespoons vegetable broth
- ➢ 1 tablespoon rice vinegar
- ➢ 1 tablespoon sesame oil, divided
- ➢ 1 teaspoon honey
- ➢ ⅛ teaspoon red chili flakes
- ➢ 2 tablespoons vegetable oil, divided
- ➢ 1 tablespoon minced garlic
- ➢ 2 teaspoons minced ginger
- ➢ ¼ cup thinly sliced green onions, white and green parts
- ➢ ¼ teaspoon sesame seeds

INSTRUCTIONS

1. Rinse the bok choy with water.
2. Shaking off any excess water and then dry using a kitchen towel or paper towels.
3. Cut each bok choy, halved lengthwise. In a small bowl combine soy sauce, broth, vinegar, 2 teaspoons of sesame oil, honey, and red chili flakes.
4. In a wok or 12-inch nonstick skillet add 1 tablespoon vegetable oil and 1 teaspoon of sesame oil over high heat until just smoking. Use tongs to carefully place the bok choy cut side down in a single layer in the wok, lightly press down to make contact with the surface.
5. Cook until lightly browned without moving, about 1 to 2 minutes. Flip the bok choy over and cook the other side until lightly browned for 1 to 2 minutes.
6. Transfer to a plate.
7. Add 1 tablespoon vegetable oil to the wok. Add garlic, ginger, and green onions, stir fry until fragrant, about 30 seconds. Add the soy sauce mixture to the wok, simmer until thickened, about 30 seconds.
8. Add bok choy back to the wok, stir-fry, and cook until the sauce glazes the greens, about 1 to 2 minutes.
9. Transfer to a platter and garnish with sesame seeds.

Cucumber Salad

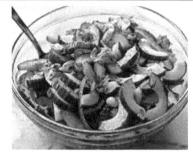

Prep Time: 15 mins **Cook Time:** 0 mins **Total Time:** 15 mins

MAKES 6 SERVINGS

INGREDIENTS

- ➤ 5 cucumbers
- ➤ 1 red onion
- ➤ 1 cup apple cider vinegar (or white vinegar, red wine vinegar, rice vinegar)
- ➤ 1/2 cup sugar (or more to taste)
- ➤ 1/2 cup water
- ➤ 1 teaspoon salt

INSTRUCTIONS

1. Peel and slice cucumbers into thin slices.
2. Cut the onion in half and cut into very thin slices.
3. Combine onions and cucumbers in a large bowl. In a separate, medium-sized bowl, combine the remaining

ingredients.

4. Stir until sugar dissolves. Pour vinegar mixture over cucumbers and onions.

5. Stir until the cucumbers are evenly coated in the dressing. Refrigerate for at least 20 minutes.

6. Before serving, drain liquid and place it in a serving bowl to serve.

Skewered Shrimp with Leeks and Yellow Squash

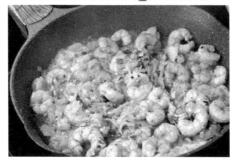

Prep Time: 15 mins **Cook Time:** 20 mins **Total Time:** 35 mins

MAKES 4 SERVINGS

INGREDIENTS

- ➢ 2 pounds wild-caught shrimp, raw, peeled & deveined
- ➢ 2 large leeks, washed, trimmed, and cut into 1/2" chunks
- ➢ 2 small, thinner yellow squash, washed, trimmed, and cut into
- ➢ 1/2" chunks
- ➢ 1 Tablespoon of tarragon, chives, garlic, lemon, salt, pepper, garlic, and onion)
- ➢ 1/2 Tablespoons Stacey Hawkins Luscious Lemon or Roasted Garlic Oil
- ➢ 8 T fresh grated Parmesan cheese for garnish
- ➢ Natural Sea salt & freshly cracked peppercorns to taste

INSTRUCTIONS

1. Preheat outdoor grill or oven to 375 degrees. Add the shrimp and veggies to a large bowl.
2. Drizzle with oil and seasonings. Toss to coat.
3. Let sit for 10 minutes, up to all day (refrigerated) to let the flavors develop. Skewer shrimp and veggies individually, or pour into a grill basket.
4. Cook for 20-25 minutes, using a spatula to turn the pieces at least once during cooking.
5. Cook until shrimp is opaque and fully cooked and vegetables are crisp-tender.
6. Serve hot, sprinkled with fresh grated Parmesan cheese for a garnish.

Thai Chicken Satay with Peanut Sauce

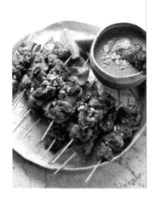

Prep Time: 40 mins **Cook Time:** 10 mins **Total Time:** 50 mins

MAKES 4 SERVINGS

INGREDIENTS

For the Chicken Satay Sauce:

- ➢ 1/2 pounds chicken tenders
- ➢ 1 cup unsweetened coconut milk
- ➢ tablespoons brown sugar
- ➢ tablespoons fish sauce
- ➢ 1 tablespoon ground coriander
- ➢ 1 teaspoon cumin
- ➢ 1/2 teaspoon turmeric
- ➢ 1 teaspoon salt Wooden Skewers, soaked

For the Peanut Dipping Sauce:

- ➢ 1/2 cup peanut butter
- ➢ 1 tablespoon fresh minced ginger
- ➢ 1/3 cup chicken broth
- ➢ 1 tablespoon honey
- ➢ 1/4 cup low-sodium soy sauce
- ➢ tablespoons rice vinegar
- ➢ 3 tablespoons sesame oil
- ➢ 2 cloves garlic 1
- ➢ tablespoon chile-garlic sauce, optional

INSTRUCTIONS

1. Combine the coconut milk, brown sugar, fish sauce, and spices in a large zip lock bag.
2. Shake and add the chicken tenders.
3. Marinate for at least 30 minutes. Soak the skewers in water for at least 30 minutes.
4. Preheat the grill to direct medium heat.
5. Weave each tender onto a skewer and lay it on a foil-covered cookie sheet.
6. Grill the Thai chicken satay for 3 minutes per side.
7. Meanwhile, puree all the ingredients for the peanut sauce in the blender and set aside.

Stuffed Eggplant

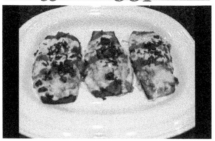

Prep Time: 15 mins **Cook Time:** 40 mins **Total Time:** 55 mins

MAKES 4 SERVINGS

INGREDIENTS

- 2 small eggplants
- Natural sea salt
- 4 tsp Stacey Hawkins Roasted Garlic Oil (or fresh garlic and oil of your choice)
- 2 lb lean ground turkey
- 1 T (one capful) Simply Brilliant Seasoning (or garlic, onion, parsley, lemon, and paprika)
- 1 C fresh tomatoes, diced (or canned, drained well)
- ½ C mushrooms, sliced
- 1 C chicken stock, preferably low sodium

INSTRUCTIONS

1. Preheat oven to 350 degrees.
2. Cut eggplants into halves, lengthwise.

3. Using a small spoon, scoop out the seeds and throw them away

4. Heat Garlic Oil in a large skillet until sizzling. Add turkey and diced eggplant.

5. Cook for 3-5 minutes, stirring occasionally until turkey is opaque. Stir in Garlic Gusto seasoning and remaining vegetables and cook for an additional minute.

6. Rinse eggplant halves to remove the salt. Pat them dry and place hollow side up in a baking dis big enough to hold all 4 halves (or use 2 baking dishes).

7. Scoop turkey mixture equally into eggplant shells.

8. Pour the stock into the bottom of the pan (use an additional cup if using 2 baking dishes) and place it on the middle rack in the oven.

9. Bake for 30-40 minutes until eggplant is fork-tender.

Keto Taco Stuffed Peppers

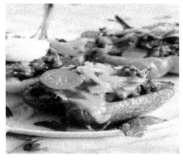

Prep Time: 10 mins **Cook Time:** 1hr **Total Time:** 1 hr 10 mins

MAKES 4 SERVINGS

INGREDIENTS

- ➢ 1 tablespoon butter
- ➢ ½ cup chopped onion
- ➢ 1 pound ground beef
- ➢ 1 taco seasoning packet look for one without fillers
- ➢ 10 ounce Rotel diced tomatoes and green chiles
- ➢ 2 cups shredded Mexican cheese blend divided
- ➢ 2 extra-large bell peppers any color (or 3 large peppers)
- ➢ Optional Toppings: Pico de gallo cilantro, sour cream, lime wedges, shredded lettuce

INSTRUCTIONS

1. Preheat the oven to 400 degrees F.
2. Cut the bell peppers in half and remove the seeds.

3. Place the pepper halves, cut side up, in a rimmed baking dish. Set a large skillet over medium heat.

4. Add the butter and onions. Sauté for 2-3 minutes to soften. Then add in the ground beef.

5. Break the meat apart with a wooden spoon and brown for 4-5 minutes. Mix in the taco seasoning, Rotel, and 1 ¼ cups shredded cheese. Stir well. Scoop the meat filling into the empty bell pepper halves.

6. Cover the dish with foil and bake for 30 minutes, or until the peppers are soft. Remove the foil for the last 5 minutes, and sprinkle the remaining cheese over the tops.

7. Serve warm, as-is, or topped with sour cream, pico de gallo, cilantro, lime wedges, or shredded lettuce.

Baked Chicken Breast

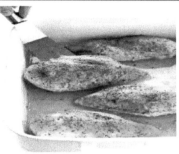

Prep Time: 5 mins **Cook Time:** 35 mins **Total Time:** 40 mins

MAKES 6 SERVINGS

INGREDIENTS

- ➢ 2 lbs boneless & skinless chicken breasts
- ➢ 1 tbsp avocado or olive oil
- ➢ 1 tsp smoked paprika
- ➢ 1 tsp garlic powder 1 tsp oregano
- ➢ 1/2 tsp salt

INSTRUCTIONS

1. Preheat oven to 450 degrees F.
2. In a medium baking dish, place chicken, drizzle with oil and sprinkle with smoked paprika, garlic powder, oregano, salt, and pepper.
3. Using tongs or hands, move the chicken around to coat on all sides evenly. Bake for 25 minutes to 35 minutes or until

150 degrees F internal temperature.

4. Remove from the oven, cover with foil or lid, and let rest for 10 minutes for the juices to settle.

5. Slice against the grain and serve along any side with a salad.

6. Meal prep for the week, use in salads and casseroles.

Orange Roast Chicken

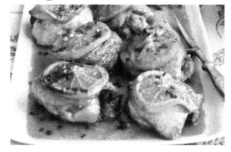

Prep Time: 10 mins **Cook Time:** 2 hr **Total Time:** 2 hr 10 mins

MAKES 4 SERVINGS

INGREDIENTS

- ➢ 7-8 pound chicken, whole
- ➢ 1/2 cup unsalted butter, softened
- ➢ 1/4 cup honey 1 small orange, such as a clementine
- ➢ Salt and pepper

For the Honey Orange Gravy:

- ➢ Pan juices from the chicken
- ➢ 3 tablespoons flour
- ➢ 2 cups chicken stock
- ➢ Salt and pepper

For The Grilled Spring Veggies:

- ➢ 12 ounces thin french green beans (haricot vert)

trimmed

- ➢ 12 ounces thin baby asparagus, trimmed
- ➢ Salt and pepper

INSTRUCTIONS

1. Preheat the oven to 450 degrees F.
2. Remove the neck and gizzards from inside the chicken. Place the chicken in a small dry skillet and pat the skin dry with paper towels. Slide a regular tablespoon, curved side down, underneath the skin of the chicken.
3. Run the spoon along the breast to loosen the skin on both sides, and down over the drumsticks.
4. Then mix the butter, honey, and the zest of one orange with 3/4 teaspoon salt and 1/4 teaspoon black pepper.
5. Mash the ingredients in a small bowl until well combined. Use the spoon to deposit the butter mixture underneath the skin of the chicken.
6. Place as much of the butter as possible over the breast meat and drumsticks. Then press the skin to smooth.
7. Rub any remaining butter over the outside of the skin and sprinkle with salt and pepper.
8. Slice the orange and place it inside the chicken. Roast the chicken for 45 minutes to crisp up the skin, then lower the heat to 350 degrees F. If the skin is brown, cover the chicken loosely with foil and continue roasting for another

75 - 90 minutes.

9. To test the chicken for doneness, stick a knife down between the drumstick and the breast.

10. If the juices run out clear, the chicken is ready. Remove the chicken from the oven and carefully lift it out of the juices.

11. Place it on a platter and cover with foil to keep it warm. While the chicken is roasting, place a large grill pan over two burners and turn them both on medium heat.

12. Lay the asparagus and green beans on the grill pan and sear until the color has intensified and grill marks have formed. Flip once and salt and pepper.

13. Cook the veggies until just cooked through, so they are bright green and firm. Approximately 6-10 minutes.

14. Place the sauté pan with the chicken juices over another burner. Heat the burner to medium heat and whisk in the flour. Add the chicken stock, then salt and pepper to taste. Bring the gravy to a boil and whisk.

15. Continue simmering and stirring until the gravy is thick enough to coat a spoon.

16. To Serve: Cut the chicken into pieces and distribute it onto plates. Spoon the grilled veggies next to the chicken and drizzle honey orange gravy over both the chicken and veggies.

Hungarian Mushroom Soup

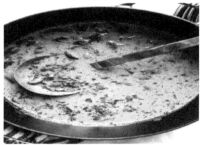

Prep Time: 15 mins **Cook Time:** 40 mins   **Total Time:** 55 mins

MAKES 6 SERVINGS

INGREDIENTS

- ¼ cups butter
- 1 large onion peeled and chopped
- 1 cup chopped celery
- 1 pound button mushrooms sliced
- 3 tablespoons soy sauce
- 2 tablespoons fresh chopped dill
- 1 tablespoon smoked paprika
- 1 tablespoon lemon juice
- 6 cups vegetable broth or mushroom broth
- ¾ cups sour cream
- 3 tablespoons all-purpose flour (or GF baking mix)
- Salt and pepper
- Garnishes: Fresh chopped dill, scallions, and/or parsley, sour cream, or cashew cream

INSTRUCTIONS

1. Set a large 6-quart saucepot over medium heat.

2. Add the butter, onions, and celery.

3. Sauté for 3-5 minutes to soften. Then move the veggies to the side of the pot and add in the mushrooms, 1 teaspoon salt, and ½ teaspoon pepper.

4. Sauté another 8-10 minutes, stirring regularly. Stir in the soy sauce, dill, smoked paprika, lemon juice, and vegetable broth. Simmer for 10-15 minutes.

5. Meanwhile, set out a medium bowl. Add the sour cream and flour. Stir until smooth. Ladle some of the soup broth into the sour cream mixture, stirring constantly so the sour cream doesn't curdle.

6. Once the mixture is thin, whisk the sour cream mixture into the soup base, whisking continually.

7. Simmer another 3-5 minutes to thicken. Taste, then add additional salt and lemon juice if needed.

8. Serve warm with a sprinkling of fresh herbs and a dollop of sour cream on top.

Crispy Brussel Sprouts

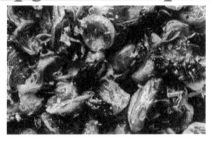

Prep Time: 15 mins **Cook Time:** 30 mins **Total Time:** 45 mins

MAKES 6 SERVINGS

INGREDIENTS

- ➢ 1/4 cup dried lentils, choose a more firm lentil type
- ➢ 2/3 cup dried quinoa
- ➢ 3 cups water
- ➢ 3/4 teaspoon curry powder
- ➢ 8 ounces Brussels sprouts
- ➢ 1 cup thinly sliced shallots,
- ➢ 2 tablespoons olive oil
- ➢ 1/2 cup Peppers,
- ➢ chopped 1/2 cup scallions, chopped
- ➢ 1/2 lemon, juiced
- ➢ Salt and pepper

INSTRUCTIONS

1. Preheat the oven to 400 degrees F.

2. Place the quinoa and lentils in a medium stockpot with 3 cups of water, 1 teaspoon salt, and 3/4 teaspoon curry powder.

3. Bring to a boil, then cover and reduce the heat to medium-low.

4. Cook for 25-30 minutes until the quinoa is fluffy and the lentils are cooked, but firm.

5. Remove from heat, but keep covered until ready to use.

6. Meanwhile, cut the Brussels sprouts in half and slice thin. Place them on a rimmed baking sheet with the sliced shallots and drizzle with olive oil. Toss to coat then spread them out thin and salt and pepper. Bake for 20-25 minutes, until crispy.

7. Fluff the quinoa and lentils and move to a large bowl.

8. Add the crispy Brussels sprouts and shallots, chopped sweet peppers, chopped scallions, and the juice of half a lemon.

9. Toss and salt and pepper to taste. Serve immediately.

Bean Salad

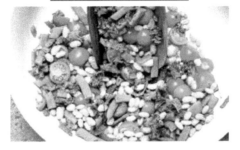

Prep Time: 15 mins **Cook Time:** 40 mins **Total Time:** 55 mins

MAKES 6 SERVINGS

INGREDIENTS

- ➢ 1 pound black-eyed peas, raw or frozen
- ➢ 1/2 pound white acre peas raw or frozen
- ➢ 1/2 pound mixed sprouted peas and lentils
- ➢ 1-pint ripe cherry tomatoes
- ➢ 1/2 small red onion, chopped
- ➢ 2 cloves garlic, minced
- ➢ 1/3 cup flat-leaf parsley, chopped
- ➢ 2 tablespoons apple cider vinegar
- ➢ 1/4 cup extra virgin olive oil
- ➢ Salt and pepper

INSTRUCTIONS

1. Place a large pot of water over high heat and bring to a boil.
2. Salt the water liberally, then add the black-eyed peas.

3. Simmer for 10 minutes, then add the white acre peas and simmer another 20-30 minutes, until both are soft and tender.

4. Drain the peas in a colander and rinse under cold water to bring the temperature down. Shake to remove excess water.

5. Place the cooked peas (beans) in a large mixing bowl.

6. Add the sprouted peas, red onion, garlic, parsley, vinegar, and oil. Toss, then salt and pepper to taste and toss again.

7. Cut the large cherry tomatoes in half and leave the small tomatoes whole. When ready to serve, pour the bean salad out on a serving platter then top with the cherry tomatoes.

Chicken Gyro Salad

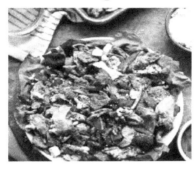

Prep Time: 30 mins **Cook Time:** 15 mins **Total Time:** 45

MAKES 4 SERVINGS

INGREDIENTS

For The Tzatziki Sauce:

- ➢ 1 cup plain Greek yogurt
- ➢ 1 hothouse cucumber
- ➢ 1 lemon, zested
- ➢ 1 tablespoon juice
- ➢ 1 tablespoon olive oil
- ➢ 1 clove garlic, minced 1 tablespoon fresh chopped dill
- ➢ 1/2 teaspoon salt
- ➢ 1/4 teaspoon pepper

For the Chicken:

- ➢ 1 pound boneless skinless chicken breast

- ➤ 1 tablespoon red wine vinegar
- ➤ 2 tablespoons olive oil
- ➤ 1 clove garlic, minced
- ➤ 1 teaspoon dried oregano
- ➤ 1/2 teaspoon crushed dried rosemary Salt and pepper

For The Salad:

- ➤ 2 pieces flatbread
- ➤ 1 cup fresh mint leaves
- ➤ 1 small red onion, sliced thin
- ➤ 1 cup sliced cucumber
- ➤ 1 cup sliced tomato wedges
- ➤ 6 cups chopped romaine lettuce

INSTRUCTIONS

1. Preheat the grill to high heat.
2. Place the chicken in a baking dish and top with vinegar, oil, herbs, 1/2 teaspoon salt, and pepper to taste.
3. Mix to coat and allow the chicken to marinate for at least 15 minutes.

For the Tzatziki Sauce:

1. Cut the cucumber in half. Use half for the tzatziki sauce and slice the remaining half for the salad.
2. Peel half of the cucumber for the tzatziki sauce and grate

it with a cheese grater.

3. Wrap the shredded cucumber in a paper towel and squeeze it firmly over the sink to extract extra moisture.

4. Then place the cumber in a bowl. Add the yogurt, zest on 1 lemon, 1 tablespoon lemon juice, olive oil, garlic, dill, salt, and pepper.

5. Mix well and refrigerate until ready to serve. Once the grill is hot, lower the heat to medium and grill the chicken for approximately 5 minutes per side. Remove the chicken and allow it to rest 5 minutes before cutting.

For the Salad:

1. Pile chopped romaine in 4 bowls.

2. Cut the flatbread into wedges.

3. Slice the chicken and layer on top of each salad.

4. Then arrange mint, red onion, cucumbers, tomato, flatbread wedges, and tzatziki sauce all around the chicken.

Egg with Muffin

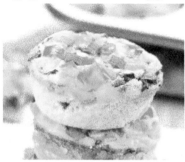

Prep Time: 15 mins **Cook Time:** 25 mins **Total Time:** 40 mins

MAKES 12 SERVINGS

INGREDIENTS

- ➢ 1 cup baby spinach, chopped
- ➢ 1/2 cup diced bell peppers
- ➢ 1/2 cup baby tomatoes, diced
- ➢ 2 cups egg whites
- ➢ 1/2 cup cottage cheese
- ➢ 1/2 teaspoon kosher salt
- ➢ 1/2 teaspoon black pepper
- ➢ 1/2 teaspoon garlic powder

INSTRUCTIONS

1. Pre-heat oven to 300°F.
2. Coat a 12-cup muffin tray with cooking spray.
3. Combine all prepared veggies in a medium mixing bowl

and then evenly divide the veggie mixture amongst the 12 muffin cups.

4. Combine egg whites, cottage cheese, salt, pepper, and garlic powder in a blender and blend until light and frothy.

5. Pour the egg mixture over the veggies, again, doing your best to divide the eggs as evenly as possible amongst all 12 muffin cups.

6. Place tray in the oven and bake for 25 minutes or until the eggs have fluffed up and are cooked through.

7. Cool before removing from the pan. They should pop out easily if you greased your pan well.

8. Serve immediately or pop into the fridge or freezer.

9. To reheat, microwave the muffins for 45-60 seconds or until thawed.

Spinach Quiche

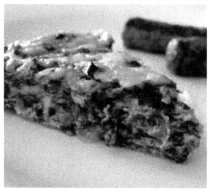

Prep Time: 5 mins **Cook Time:** 20 mins **Total Time:** 25 mins

MAKES 4 SERVINGS

INGREDIENTS

- ➢ 1 tablespoon olive oil
- ➢ 4-8 ounces white mushrooms, sliced
- ➢ 1 clove garlic, minced
- ➢ 10 oz box frozen spinach, thawed and squeezed dry
- ➢ 6 eggs 3/4 cup milk,
- ➢ 3/4 cup heavy cream
- ➢ 1/3 cup sharp cheddar, diced
- ➢ 3/4 cup shredded Gouda cheese
- ➢ Salt and pepper to taste
- ➢ 3/4 teaspoon kosher salt
- ➢ 1/4 teaspoon black pepper

INSTRUCTIONS

1. Preheat the oven to 350°F.

2. Grease a 9-inch pie plate and set it aside.

3. Add olive oil to a non-stick skillet and saute the mushrooms, garlic, and a pinch of salt until mushrooms are lightly browned and have given off all their liquid.

4. Add the spinach and mix and heat for a minute to remove any excess moisture.

5. Place the spinach mixture in the bottom of the pie dish, followed by the cheddar chunks. In a medium bowl, whisk together the eggs, milk, cream, salt, and pepper.

6. Pour the egg mixture into the pie plate. Top with the shredded Gouda cheese.

7. Bake for 45-55 minutes, or until the top is golden brown.

8. Slice and serve

Cloud Bread

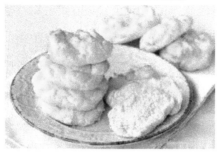

Prep Time: 15 mins **Cook Time:** 20 mins **Total Time:** 35 mins

MAKES 10 SERVINGS

INGREDIENTS

- ➢ 4 large eggs, separated
- ➢ 1/2 teaspoon cream of tartar
- ➢ 2 ounces low-fat cream cheese
- ➢ 1 teaspoon Italian herb seasoning
- ➢ 1/2 teaspoon sea salt
- ➢ 1/2 teaspoon garlic powder

INSTRUCTIONS

1. Preheat the oven to 300 degrees F.
2. If you have a convection oven, set it on convect. Line two large baking sheets with parchment paper.
3. Separate the egg whites and egg yolks. Place the whites in a stand mixer with a whip attachment.

4. Add the cream of tartar and beat on high until the froth turns into firm meringue peaks. Move to a separate bowl.

5. Place the cream cheese in the empty stand mixing bowl. Beat on high to soften.

6. Then add the egg yolks one at a time to incorporate. Scrape the bowl and beat until the mixture is completely smooth.

7. Then beat in the Italian seasoning, salt, and garlic powder. Gently fold the firm meringue into the yolk mixture.

8. Try to deflate the meringue as little as possible, so the mixture is still firm and foamy.

9. Spoon 1/4 cup portions of the foam onto the baking sheets and spread into even 4-inch circles, 3/4 inch high.

10. Make sure to leave space around each circle. Bake on convect for 15-18 minutes, or in a conventional oven for up to 30 minutes. The bread should be golden on the outside and firm.

11. The center should not jiggle when shaken.

12. Cool for several minutes on the baking sheets, then move and serve

Zucchini Shrimp Scampi

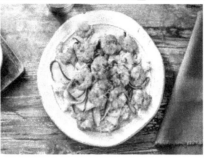

Prep Time: 15 mins **Cook Time:** 15 mins **Total Time:** 30mins

MAKES 4 SERVINGS

INGREDIENTS

- ➤ 2 tablespoons unsalted butter
- ➤ 1 pound medium shrimp, peeled and deveined
- ➤ 3 cloves garlic, minced
- ➤ 1/2 teaspoon red pepper flakes, or more, to taste
- ➤ 1/4 cup chicken stock Juice of 1 lemon
- ➤ salt and black pepper, to taste
- ➤ 1/2 pounds zucchini, spiralized
- ➤ 2 tablespoons freshly grated Parmesan
- ➤ 2 tablespoons chopped fresh parsley leaves

INSTRUCTIONS

1. Melt butter in a large skillet over medium-high heat.
2. Add shrimp, garlic, and red pepper flakes.

3. Cook, stirring occasionally, until pink, about 2-3 minutes.
4. Stir in chicken stock and lemon juice; season with salt and pepper, to taste.
5. Bring to a simmer; stir in zucchini noodles until well combined, about 1-2 minutes. Serve immediately, garnished with Parmesan and parsley, if desired.

Spinach Artichoke Dip

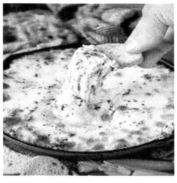

Prep Time: 5 mins **Cook Time:** 25 mins **Total Time:** 30 mins

MAKES 8 SERVINGS

INGREDIENTS

- ➢ 8 ounces reduced-fat cream cheese room temperature
- ➢ ½ cup plain non-fat Greek yogurt
- ➢ ½ cup sour cream full-fat or reduced-fat
- ➢ 10 ounces frozen spinach defrosted and drained
- ➢ ½ cup jarred artichokes drained and chopped
- ➢ ¼ cup freshly grated Parmesan cheese
- ➢ ⅓ cup shredded Mozzarella Cheese
- ➢ ⅓ cup Feta cheese crumbled
- ➢ 2 teaspoons minced garlic
- ➢ ¼ teaspoon crushed red pepper flakes optional
- ➢ 1 teaspoon fresh lemon juice
- ➢ ½ teaspoon kosher salt

INSTRUCTIONS

1. Preheat oven to 350 degrees and grease a 1-quart baking dish.

2. Defrost frozen spinach in the microwave or overnight in the refrigerator. Place defrosted spinach in cheesecloth or clean kitchen towel and squeeze out excess moisture over the sink.

3. Drain a 10-ounce jar of artichoke hearts and chop well, measure out ½ cup of artichokes to use for the dip. In a large mixing bowl cream the cream cheese, sour cream, and yogurt together until creamy and smooth.

4. Add the spinach, artichokes, cheese, salt, lemon juice, garlic cloves, and red pepper flakes to the cream cheese mixture and mix until all the ingredients are well incorporated.

5. Transfer the mixture to the greased baking dish.

6. Bake at 350 degrees for 20-25 minutes or until warmed through and slightly browned on the top.

7. Serve with veggies, tortilla chips, or pita chips.

Keto Meatloaf

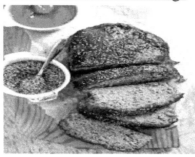

Prep Time: 10 mins **Cook Time:** 1 hr 25 mins **Total Time:** 1 hr 35 mins

MAKES 8 SERVINGS

INGREDIENTS

- ➢ 2 pounds 80/20 Ground beef
- ➢ 1 medium Onion, diced
- ➢ 2 cups Crushed Pork rinds
- ➢ 1 large Egg
- ➢ 2 tablespoons Worcestershire sauce
- ➢ ½ teaspoon Garlic powder
- ➢ 1 teaspoon salt
- ➢ ⅓ cup Reduced sugar ketchup

INSTRUCTIONS

1. Preheat oven to 350 degrees F.
2. In a large bowl combine all ingredients except ketchup.
3. Mix ingredients until fully combined.

4. Press ingredients into a parchment paper-lined loaf pan. Bake for 30 minutes.
5. After 30 minutes add ketchup on top and bake for 25-35 minutes more.
6. Remove from oven and let rest for 15 minutes.

Spaghetti Squash Lasagna

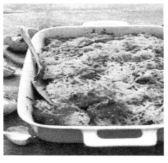

Prep Time: 10 mins **Cook Time:** 1hr **Total Time:** 1 hr 10 mins

MAKES 6 SERVINGS

INGREDIENTS

- ➢ 2 medium spaghetti squash
- ➢ 1 tablespoon plus
- ➢ 2 teaspoons olive oil divided
- ➢ 2 teaspoons kosher salt divided
- ➢ ¾ teaspoon black pepper divided
- ➢ 1 pound ground turkey
- ➢ 2 teaspoons Italian seasoning
- ➢ ¼ teaspoon red pepper flakes
- ➢ 2 cloves garlic minced
- ➢ 1 (24-ounce) jar good-quality tomato pasta sauce I like roasted garlic
- ➢ 1 tablespoon red wine vinegar
- ➢ 1 (10-ounce) pack frozen spinach drained

- ➢ 1 cup part-skim ricotta cheese
- ➢ 1 cup shredded fontina, mild provolone, mozzarella, or similar melty cheese divided
- ➢ ¼ cup grated Parmesan cheese

INSTRUCTIONS

1. Place a rack in the center of your oven and preheat the oven to 400 degrees F.
2. Roast the spaghetti squash according to this recipe for Roasted Spaghetti Squash.
3. While the squash is baking, heat the remaining tablespoon of oil in a large skillet over medium-high.
4. Add the turkey, 1 teaspoon salt, remaining ½ teaspoon pepper, Italian seasoning, and red pepper flakes. Stir and cook, breaking apart the meat into small pieces, until it is fully cooked through and browned on all sides, about 4 minutes.
5. Stir in the garlic and cook until fragrant, about 1 minute more. Reduce the heat to low. Stir in the pasta sauce and red wine vinegar. Let simmer for 1 minute.
6. Taste and adjust the seasoning as desired. Place the spinach in a large mixing bowl.
7. Use a fork to separate any large clumps. Add the ricotta, ½ cup fontina, and remaining ½ teaspoon salt.
8. Stir with the fork to combine. When the squash is cool

enough to handle, use a fork to fluff the insides into strands and add the strands to the bowl. With the same fork, stir to combine, evenly distributing the ingredients as best you can.

9. Return the squash halves to the baking sheet, cut sides up. Fill the squash: Pile the ricotta/squash filling evenly into each of the four halves. Top with tomato sauce, remaining shredded cheese, and Parmesan.

10. Return to the oven and bake until the filling is fully heated through and the cheese is melty about 10 to 15 minutes.

11. Brown the top (optional): Turn the oven to broil. Broil the squash until the cheese is extra bubbly and lightly browned, about 2 minutes.

12. Watch it carefully, and do not walk away so that it doesn't burn. Sprinkle with parsley and enjoy!

Zucchini Lasagna

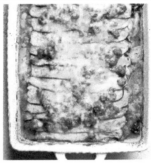

Prep Time: 30 mins **Cook Time:** 20 **Total Time:** 50 mins

MAKES 8 SERVINGS

INGREDIENTS

- ➤ 2 medium zucchini
- ➤ 1 pound beef, ground
- ➤ 1/2 medium onion
- ➤ 1/2 medium bell pepper, red
- ➤ 2 medium carrot
- ➤ 3 clove garlic
- ➤ 15-ounce tomato sauce
- ➤ 1 tablespoon Worcestershire sauce
- ➤ 1 teaspoon oregano, dried
- ➤ 1 teaspoon basil, dried
- ➤ 1/8 teaspoon salt
- ➤ 1/8 teaspoon black pepper, ground
- ➤ 2 cup cottage cheese

- ➤ 1 large egg
- ➤ 1/4 cup Parmesan cheese, grated
- ➤ 2 cup mozzarella cheese

INSTRUCTIONS

1. Wash and cut zucchini into very thin strips.
2. Line a colander with paper towels and place it in the sink. Place zucchini into the colander and salt generously.
3. Allow zucchini strips to sweat for 30 minutes.
4. Dice onion and red bell pepper (enough for 1/2 cup), grated carrots (enough for 1/2 cup), and mince garlic. Pre-heat oven to 350* F and grease a 9×13 inch pan. In a large skillet over medium-high heat, brown ground beef until cooked completely, making sure to chop into small pieces as you go.
5. Remove beef onto a paper towel-lined plate and set aside. Remove most of the remaining fat from the skillet, place it back on the stove, and saute the onion, pepper, carrot, and garlic until the onion is translucent.
6. Add tomato sauce, Worcestershire sauce, spices, and the cooked ground beef back into the skillet.
7. Bring to a simmer, and allow to simmer for 10 minutes. Meanwhile, mix cottage cheese, egg, and parmesan in a small bowl. Once the zucchini have sweat for 30 minutes, wipe clean and dry with a clean cloth.

8. Place one layer of zucchini strips on the bottom of the greased pan. On top of the zucchini, spread half of the tomato-beef sauce. Then spread a layer of half of the cottage cheese mixture.

9. Then sprinkle half of the mozzarella cheese. Repeat layers once more: zucchini, sauce, cottage cheese, mozzarella.

10. Place in the oven for 20 minutes at 350* F, then turn the oven to broil and crack the oven door.

11. Allow the top of the lasagna to bubble and brown, watching carefully. Should take 2 minutes or less.

12. Remove from the oven and allow to sit for 20-30 minutes before serving.

Salmon Florentine

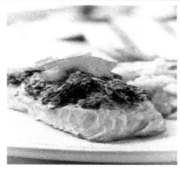

Prep Time: 15 mins **Cook Time:** 10 mins **Total Time:** 25 mins

MAKES 4 SERVINGS

INGREDIENTS

- ➤ 2 (10 ounce) packages frozen spinach
- ➤ 1 tablespoon olive oil
- ➤ 1/4 cup minced shallots
- ➤ 2 teaspoons minced garlic
- ➤ 5 sun-dried tomatoes, chopped
- ➤ 1/4 teaspoon red pepper flakes
- ➤ 1/2 teaspoon salt
- ➤ 1/4 teaspoon black pepper
- ➤ 1/2 cup part-skim ricotta cheese
- ➤ 4 (6-ounce) salmon fillets

INSTRUCTIONS

1. Preheat oven to 350 degrees F.

2. Using your hands, squeeze spinach of all excess liquid.

3. Heat olive oil in a large skillet over medium heat. Add shallots and garlic and cook for 3 minutes until they begin to soften.

4. Add garlic and cook for 1 minute more.

5. Add spinach, sun-dried tomatoes, red pepper flakes, 1/2 teaspoon salt, and 1/4 teaspoon pepper, and cook an additional 2 minutes. Remove from heat and let cool for approximately 10 minutes. Add ricotta and stir to combine.

6. Season with additional salt and pepper, to taste. Using your hands, pack approximately 1/2 cup spinach mixture on top of each salmon fillet, forming mixture to the shape of the fillet.

7. Place fillets on a rimmed baking sheet or glass baking dish and bake for 15 minutes, until salmon is cooked through.

Zucchini Chips

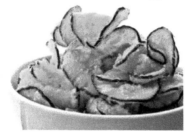

Prep Time: 10 mins **Cook Time:** 50 mins **Total Time:** 1hr

MAKES 3 SERVINGS

INGREDIENTS

- ➤ 1 medium zucchini washed and dried
- ➤ 1 tbsp. olive oil Scant
- ➤ ½ tsp. kosher salt
- ➤ ½ tsp. black pepper
- ➤ ¼ tsp. onion powder
- ➤ ½ tsp. paprika

INSTRUCTIONS

1. Preheat the oven to 450 degrees.
2. Line two baking sheets with parchment paper. Thinly slice the zucchini with a knife or mandolin.
3. In a large bowl, combine the oil, salt, pepper, onion powder, and paprika. Stir to combine.
4. Add the zucchini slices to the bowl and toss well so that

each slice is coated with the seasoned oil. Place the zucchini slices on the prepared baking sheets.

5. Bake for 8-15 minutes watching very closely. When the zucchini starts to show some brown spots remove from the oven and set aside.

6. Reduce the oven temperature to 180-200 degrees. Return the zucchini to the oven and cook for an additional 20-40 minutes or until the slices are crispy.

7. Remove from the oven and cool.

Homemade Spaghetti Souce

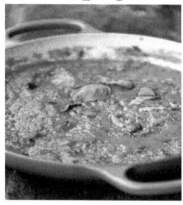

Prep Time: 15 mins **Cook Time:** 50 mins **Total Time:** 1hr 5 mins

MAKES 10 SERVINGS

INGREDIENTS

- ➢ 1 1/2 pounds ground beef
- ➢ 3 teaspoons minced garlic
- ➢ 2 cans tomato puree
- ➢ 29 ounces each
- ➢ 2 cans diced tomatoes, with juice 14.5 ounces each
- ➢ 2 teaspoons salt
- ➢ 2 teaspoons lemon juice
- ➢ 2 tablespoons olive oil
- ➢ 2 teaspoons oregano
- ➢ 2 teaspoons basil
- ➢ 1 teaspoon thyme
- ➢ 1 teaspoon crushed red pepper

INSTRUCTIONS

1. In a large saucepan, brown the ground beef along with the garlic. Drain.
2. Add in the rest of the ingredients and bring to a low boil, stirring often.
3. Once the sauce is heated through and at a low boil, reduce the burner temperature to low and simmer uncovered for 45 minutes.
4. Serve immediately or allow the sauce to cool, then package it in freezer-safe containers for easy storage.

Olive Oil Seared Scallops

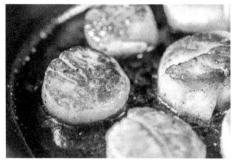

Prep Time: 5 mins **Cook Time:** 5 mins **Total Time:** 10 mins

MAKES 2 SERVINGS

INGREDIENTS

- ➤ 1 pound sea scallops
- ➤ 1/4 teaspoon kosher salt (or to taste)
- ➤ 1/4 teaspoon ground black pepper
- ➤ 2 tablespoons olive oil

INSTRUCTIONS

1. If not done in advance, remove the small side muscle from each scallop.
2. Rinse scallops under cold water and pat dry with paper towels. Season with salt and pepper.
3. Add olive oil to a large saute pan and heat on medium-high heat until the oil starts to shimmer but before it smokes.

4. Carefully add scallops to the pan, making sure there is space between each scallop.

5. Cook the scallops for about 2 minutes, flip carefully to the other side and cook for another 2 minutes. They should have a nice golden crust and still be slightly translucent on the inside.

6. Serve immediately.

Roasted Parsnips and Carrots

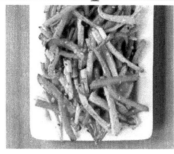

Prep Time: 15 mins **Cook Time:** 25 mins **Total Time:** 40 mins

MAKES 8 SERVINGS

INGREDIENTS

- ➢ 4 large parsnips
- ➢ 4 large carrots
- ➢ 2 tablespoons oil olive, sunflower, canola, grapeseed
- ➢ 3 teaspoons rosemary
- ➢ 2 teaspoons kosher salt
- ➢ 1 teaspoon thyme

INSTRUCTIONS

1. Preheat oven to 425 degrees.
2. Peel the parsnips and carrots.
3. Quarter the thick end of the carrots, and half them on the thinner end.
4. Quarter the parsnips. Cut out the thick, fibrous center,

then cut them the same as the carrots

5. Combine parsnips and carrots in a large bowl and toss with oil, rosemary, salt, and thyme.

Kale & Bell Frittata

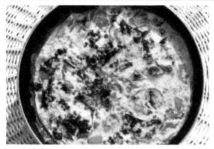

Prep Time: 15 mins **Cook Time:** 20 mins **Total Time:** 35 mins

MAKES 4 SERVINGS

INGREDIENTS

- ➢ 6 eggs Salt, as required
- ➢ 1 tablespoon olive oil
- ➢ ½ teaspoon ground turmeric
- ➢ 1 small red bell pepper, seeded and chopped
- ➢ 1 cup fresh kale, trimmed and chopped
- ➢ ¼ cup fresh chives, chopped

INSTRUCTIONS

1. In a bowl, add the eggs and salt and beat well. Set aside.
2. In a cast-iron skillet, heat the oil over medium-low heat and sprinkle with turmeric. Immediately stir in the bell pepper and kale and sauté for about 2 minutes.
3. Place the beaten eggs over bell pepper mixture evenly

and immediately reduce the heat to low.

4. Cover the skillet and cook for about 10-15 minutes.

5. Remove from the heat and set aside for about 5 minutes.

6. Cut into equal-sized wedges and serve.

Kale, Apple & Cranberry Salad

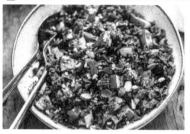

Prep Time: 15 mins **Cook Time:** 0 mins **Total Time:** 15 mins

MAKES 4 SERVINGS

INGREDIENTS

- ➢ 6 cups fresh baby kale
- ➢ 3 large apples, cored and sliced
- ➢ ¼ cup unsweetened dried cranberries
- ➢ ¼ cup almonds, sliced
- ➢ 2 tablespoons extra-virgin olive oil
- ➢ 1 tablespoon raw honey
- ➢ Salt and ground black pepper, as required

INSTRUCTIONS

1. In a salad bowl, place all the ingredients and toss to coat well.
2. Serve immediately

Spinach and Mushroom Stew

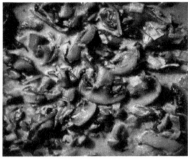

Prep Time: 15 mins **Cook Time:** 30 mins **Total Time:** 45 mins

MAKES 4 SERVINGS

INGREDIENTS

- ➢ 2 tablespoons olive oil
- ➢ 2 onions, chopped
- ➢ 3 garlic cloves, minced
- ➢ ½ pound fresh button mushrooms, chopped
- ➢ ¼ pound fresh shiitake mushrooms, chopped
- ➢ ¼ pound fresh spinach, chopped
- ➢ salt and black pepper, to taste
- ➢ ¼ cup low-sodium vegetable broth
- ➢ ½ cup coconut milk
- ➢ 2 tablespoons fresh parsley, chopped

INSTRUCTIONS

1. In a large skillet, heat oil over medium heat and sauté the

onion and garlic for 4-5 minutes.

2. Add the mushrooms, salt, and black pepper and cook for 4-5 minutes.
3. Add the spinach, broth and coconut milk and bring to a gentle boil. Simmer for 4-5 minutes or until desired doneness.
4. Stir in the cilantro and remove from heat.
5. Serve hot.

Chicken Burgers

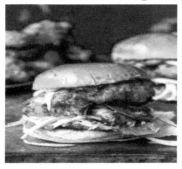

Prep Time: 15 mins **Cook Time:** 10 mins **Total Time:** 25 mins

MAKES 4 SERVINGS

INGREDIENTS

- ➢ 1¼ pounds ground chicken
- ➢ 1 egg ½ yellow onion, grated
- ➢ Salt and ground black pepper, as required
- ➢ 1 teaspoon dried thyme
- ➢ 2 tablespoons olive oil
- ➢ 4 cups lettuce, torn
- ➢ 1 cucumber, chopped

INSTRUCTIONS

1. In a bowl, add all the ingredients and mix until well combined.
2. Make 8 small equal-sized patties from the mixture.
3. In a large frying pan, heat the oil over medium heat and

cook the patties for about 4-5 minutes per side or until done completely.

4. Divide the lettuce and cucumber onto serving plates and top each with 2 burgers.

5. Serve hot.

Clam Chowder

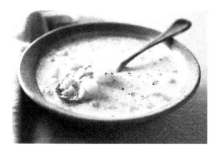

Prep Time: 10 mins **Cook Time**: 45 mins **Total Time:** 55 mins

MAKES 4 SERVINGS

INGREDIENTS

- ➤ 3 tablespoons extra-virgin olive oil
- ➤ 1 cup diced onion
- ➤ 1 cup diced celery
- ➤ ½ cup all-purpose flour
- ➤ ½ teaspoon dried thyme
- ➤ ¼ teaspoon salt
- ➤ ¼ teaspoon ground pepper
- ➤ 1 bay leaf
- ➤ 4 cups clam juice
- ➤ 1 cup whole milk
- ➤ 3 cups diced white potatoes
- ➤ 1 16-ounce container chopped fresh clams (plus their liquid), thawed if frozen Chopped cooked
- ➤ bacon for garnish Snipped chives for garnish

INSTRUCTIONS

1. Heat oil in a large pot over medium heat.
2. Add onion and celery; cook, stirring frequently until softened and beginning to brown, 3 to 6 minutes.
3. Sprinkle flour, thyme, salt, pepper, and bay leaf over the vegetables and cook, stirring, for 1 minutes more.
4. Add clam juice (or seafood stock) and milk; bring to a gentle boil, stirring constantly.
5. Stir in potatoes and bring just to a simmer.
6. Simmer, uncovered, stirring occasionally, until the potatoes are tender, 12 to 15 minutes. Add clams and cook, stirring frequently, until cooked through, 2 to 4 minutes.
7. Serve topped with bacon and chives, if desired.

Turkey Chili

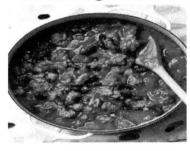

Prep Time: 15 mins **Cook Time:** 30 mins **Total Time:** 45 mins

MAKES 4 SERVINGS

INGREDIENTS

- ➢ 1 1/2 cup red bell pepper, diced
- ➢ 1 cup red onion, diced
- ➢ 1 cup celery, chopped
- ➢ 4 cloves garlic, minced 1/2 cup butter
- ➢ 6 tablespoons masa
- ➢ 2 tablespoons ground cumin
- ➢ 2 tablespoons ground coriander
- ➢ 1/2 tablespoons chili powder
- ➢ 1 tablespoon dried oregano
- ➢ 6 cups turkey stock or chicken stock
- ➢ 6 cups turkey meat, cooked and chopped
- ➢ 45 ounces canned black beans, drained and rinsed
- ➢ 1 1/2 cups frozen corn
- ➢ 2 tablespoon honey

- ➤ Salt and pepper to taste
- ➤ Possible Toppings: shredded cheese, sour cream, diced red onion, chopped scallions, salsa, corn chips

INSTRUCTIONS

1. Place the butter in a large stockpot and set over medium heat.
2. Add the bell pepper, onions, celery, and garlic. Sauté for 5-8 minutes, until softened.
3. Stir to make sure the veggies don't burn.
4. Mix in the masa, cumin, coriander, chili powder, and oregano. Stir to coat and sauté for another 2 minutes.
5. Then pour in the turkey stock and scrape the bottom of the pot to loosen the veggies.
6. Add the chopped turkey, beans, corn, and honey.
7. Season with 1 1/2 teaspoons of salt and 1/2 teaspoon ground pepper. Bring the chili to a low boil and simmer for at least 20 minutes, stirring occasionally.
8. Taste and season again if needed. Serve warm.

Harvest Salad

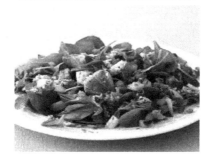

Prep Time: 20 mins **Cook Time:** 2 mins **Total Time:** 22 mins

MAKES 4 SERVINGS

INGREDIENTS

For The Cobb Salad:

➢ 2 romaine hearts roughly chopped

➢ 2 cups cooked chicken cut into cubes

➢ 2 cups roasted butternut squash cubes

➢ 6 slices thick-cut bacon cooked and crumbled

➢ 3 large hard-boiled eggs peeled and chopped

➢ 2 ripe avocadoes sliced

➢ 1 cup shelled pecans

➢ 1 tablespoon butter

➢ 1/4 teaspoon ground mustard

➢ 1/4 teaspoon garlic powder

➢ 1/4 teaspoon hot paprika

➢ 1/4 teaspoon salt

For The Creamy Corn And Poblano Dressing:

- ➢ 1 poblano pepper
- ➢ 1 clove garlic
- ➢ 2 ears corn on the cob cooked
- ➢ 2 limes juiced
- ➢ 1 teaspoon ground cumin
- ➢ 1 teaspoon salt
- ➢ 2/3 cup olive oil

<u>INSTRUCTIONS</u>

1. Heat a skillet to medium-low heat.
2. Melt the butter in the skillet, then add the pecans.
3. Sprinkle the pecans with the ground mustard, garlic powder, paprika, and salt and toss to coat. Sauté for 3-5 minutes, stirring regularly to toast. Be careful not to burn the pecans.
4. Pile the chopped romaine on a large platter.
5. Arrange the chopped chicken, roasted butternut squash, bacon, pecans, eggs, and avocados in rows on top of the romaine.
6. Preheat the oven to broil. Place the poblano pepper on a small baking sheet and set it on the top rack in the oven.
7. Check the pepper every 1-2 minutes, turning when the skin is black and blistered. Remove the poblano from the oven when it's black on all sides. Place the pepper in a zip

bag and allow it to steam for 10 minutes.

8. Cut the corn off the cobs and place them in the blender. Add the garlic clove, lime juice, salt, and cumin.

9. Once the pepper has steamed, removed the papery skin, stem, and seeds. Place the poblano flesh in the blender.

10. Puree until smooth, then remove the ingredient cup from the lid and slowly pour in the olive oil to emulsify.

11. Once the dressing is smooth and creamy, turn off the blender and pour the dressing into a serving bowl.

Bacon and Eggs

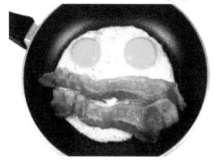

Prep Time: 2 mins **Cook Time:** 10 mins **Total Time:** 12 mins

MAKES 4 SERVINGS

INGREDIENTS

- ➤ 8 eggs
- ➤ 9 oz. bacon, in slices
- ➤ cherry tomatoes (optional)
- ➤ fresh thyme (optional)

INSTRUCTIONS

1. Fry the bacon in a pan on medium-high heat until crispy.
2. Put aside on a plate. Leave the rendered fat in the pan.
3. Use the same pan to fry the eggs. Place it over medium heat and crack your eggs into the bacon grease.
4. You can also crack them into a measuring cup and carefully pour them into the pan to avoid splattering of hot grease. Cook the eggs any way you like them.

5. For the sunny side up leave the eggs to fry on one side and cover the pan with a lid to make sure they get cooked on top.
6. For eggs cooked over easy flip the eggs over after a few minutes and cook for another minute.
7. Cut the cherry tomatoes in half and fry them at the same time.
8. Salt and pepper to taste.

Lean Green Lettuce Tacos

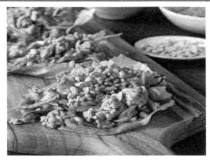

Prep Time: 15 mins **Cook Time:** 10 mins **Total Time:** 25 mins

MAKES 8 SERVINGS

INGREDIENTS

- ➢ 1 small zucchini, diced
- ➢ 1 small yellow squash, diced
- ➢ ½ pound extra-lean ground beef
- ➢ 1 tablespoon olive oil
- ➢ 1 (1.25-oz.) taco fresco seasoning
- ➢ 1 (8-oz.) can no-salt-added tomato sauce
- ➢ 2 tablespoons chopped fresh cilantro
- ➢ 1 tablespoon lime juice
- ➢ 8 romaine lettuce leaves
- ➢ Toppings: diced tomato, chopped fresh cilantro, chopped red onion, crumbled queso fresco

INSTRUCTIONS

1. Sauté first 3 ingredients in hot oil in a large nonstick skillet over medium-high heat 5 to 6 minutes or until meat crumbles and is no longer pink.
2. Stir in seasoning until blended; cook 1 minute.
3. Reduce heat to low; stir in tomato sauce, and cook, stirring often, 3 to 4 minutes or until thoroughly heated.
4. Remove from heat, and stir in cilantro and lime juice.
5. Serve meat mixture in romaine lettuce leaves with desired toppings. 2% reduced-fat shredded Cheddar or Monterey Jack cheese may be substituted.
6. Note: For testing purposes only, we used Nueva Cocina Taco Fresco Ground Beef Seasoning.

Cauliflower Rice Stuffed Peppers

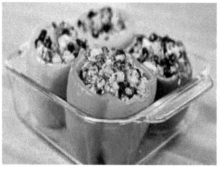

Prep Time: 1hr **Cook Time:** 40 mins **Total Time:** 1 hr 40mins

MAKES 4 SERVINGS

INGREDIENTS

- 4 large bell peppers (about 2 pounds)
- 2 cups small cauliflower florets
- 2 tablespoons extra-virgin olive oil, divided Pinch of salt plus
- 1/2 teaspoon, divided Pinch of ground pepper plus
- 1/4 teaspoon, divided
- ½ cup chopped onion
- 1 pound lean ground beef
- 2 cloves garlic, minced
- ½ teaspoon dried oregano
- 1 (8 ounces) can no-salt-added tomato sauce
- ½ cup shredded part-skim mozzarella

INSTRUCTIONS

1. Preheat oven to 350 degrees F.

2. Slice off stem ends of bell peppers.

3. Cut the flesh from the stem and chop. You should have about 1 cup. Scoop out seeds from the pepper cavities. Bring about an inch of water to a boil in a large pot fitted with a steamer basket.

4. Steam the peppers until starting to soften, about 3 minutes. Remove the peppers from the pot and set them aside.

5. Pulse cauliflower in a food processor until broken down into rice- size pieces. Heat 1 tablespoon oil in a large skillet over medium heat. Add the cauliflower rice and a pinch each of salt and pepper.

6. Cook, stirring until softened and starting to brown, about 3 minutes. Transfer to a small bowl. Wipe out the pan.

7. Add the remaining 1 tablespoon oil, the chopped bell pepper, and onion. Cook, stirring, until starting to soften, about 3 minutes.

8. Add beef, garlic, oregano, and the remaining 1/2 teaspoon salt and 1/4 teaspoon pepper.

9. Cook, stirring and breaking up the beef with a wooden spoon just until no longer pink, about 5 minutes. Add tomato sauce and the cauliflower rice; stir to coat. Place the peppers upright in an 8-inch square baking dish.

10. Fill each pepper with a generous 1 cup of the cauliflower rice mixture. Top each pepper with 2 tablespoons of cheese.
11. Bake until the filling is heated through and the cheese is melted, 20 to 25 minutes.

Cream of Thyme Soup

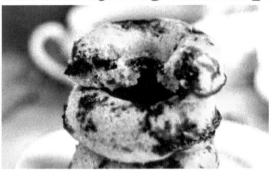

Prep Time: 5 mins **Cook Time:** 10 mins **Total Time:** 15 mins

MAKES 6 SERVINGS

INGREDIENTS

- 1 1/4 cups whole wheat pastry flour, spoon in, and level off the top
- 1 teaspoon baking powder
- 1/2 teaspoon salt
- 1/4 cup sugar
- 1 egg
- 1/2 cup milk (I like almond milk or cashew milk)
- 1 teaspoon vanilla extract
- 2 tablespoons coconut oil, melted (any oil or even melted butter will work)
- 1/2-1 cup fresh blueberries Powdered sugar, optional topping

INSTRUCTIONS

1. Pre-heat oven to 350° F.

2. In a large bowl, combine flour, baking powder, salt, and sugar. Stir in egg, milk, vanilla extract, and coconut oil. I add the coconut oil last and stir swiftly, as to avoid it hardening up.

3. Gradually, stir in blueberries. Spoon batter into a liberally greased donut pan (nonstick spray works fine).

4. You can also use a piping bag or a freezer bag with the tip snipped off to pipe the donut batter into the pan. Divide equally to create 10 donuts. The batter should fill donut molds to the center (but not cover it).

5. Bake for 9-10 minutes. Let donuts cool for about 5 minutes before removing them from the donut pan. You may need to use a knife to remove each donut from the pan.

6. To make the donut glaze, mix all glaze ingredients in a medium bowl. You may need to add a bit more water 1-2 teaspoons at a time for the right consistency.

7. Dip warm donuts into the glaze, making sure to coat both sides, if desired. Place onto wire cooling rack to allow excess glaze to drip down.

8. The glaze will eventually set + harden on the donuts after about 20 minutes.

9. Donuts are best enjoyed the same day, though they keep

at room temperature for a couple of extra days in an airtight container.

Broccoli Quiche with Cheddar

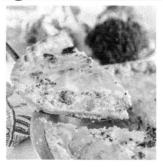

Prep Time: 10 mins **Cook Time:** 30 mins **Total Time:** 50 mins

MAKES 4 SERVINGS

INGREDIENTS

- ➤ 1 tablespoon butter for pan
- ➤ 1 (16 oz) package frozen chopped broccoli
- ➤ 8 large eggs ½ cup sour cream (or full-fat Greek yogurt)
- ➤ 1 teaspoon Diamond Cr
- ➤ ystal kosher salt
- ➤ ¼ teaspoon black pepper
- ➤ 1 teaspoon garlic powder
- ➤ ¼ cup chopped scallions white and green parts
- ➤ 1 cup shredded sharp cheddar cheese

INSTRUCTIONS

1. Preheat oven to 400 degrees F.
2. Generously butters a 9-inch pie dish.

3. Place the broccoli in a large microwave-safe bowl.

4. Add ¼ cup water. Cover and microwave on high for 6 minutes, stirring after the first 3 minutes. Drain well. In a large bowl, whisk together the eggs, sour cream, Kosher salt, black pepper, and garlic powder.

5. Stir in the broccoli, the scallions, and the cheese. Transfer the mixture to the prepared pie dish.

6. Bake until golden brown and a knife inserted in center comes out clean, about 30 minutes.

7. Allow the quiche to cool and set in pan on a wire rack, about 15 minutes, before slicing into 8 triangles and serving.

Potato Flatbread

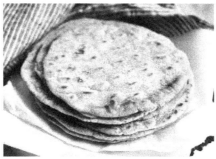

Prep Time: 15 mins **Cook Time:** 20 mins **Total Time:** 35 mins

MAKES 8 SERVINGS

INGREDIENTS

- ➢ 1 cup Mashed Potatoes (about 8.5 ounces/240 grams fresh potatoes)
- ➢ 1 cup All-Purpose Flour

INSTRUCTIONS

1. Place the flour and potato mash onto your work surface.
2. Using your hand(s) start bringing the ingredients together until you form a sticky dough. Roll this into a sausage and cut it into 8 pieces.
3. Form each piece into a round shape.
4. Make sure the worktop and dough are dusted with flour before you start rolling it out. Roll it out thin.
5. Cook on medium to high heat on a dry frying pan for

about 2 minutes (1 minute per side) or until done.

6. Best served right away while still warm.

Heavenly Halibut

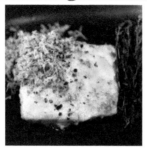

Prep Time: 20 mins **Cook Time:** 25 mins **Total Time:** 45 mins

MAKES 4 SERVINGS

INGREDIENTS

- ½ cup grated Parmesan cheese
- ¼ cup butter softened
- 3 tablespoons mayonnaise
- 2 tablespoons lemon juice
- 3 tablespoons chopped green onions
- ¼ teaspoon salt
- 1 dash hot pepper sauce
- 2 pounds skinless halibut fillets

INSTRUCTIONS

1. Preheat the oven broiler.
2. Grease a baking dish.
3. In a bowl, mix the Parmesan cheese, butter, mayonnaise,

lemon juice, green onions, salt, and hot pepper sauce.

4. Arrange the halibut fillets in the prepared baking dish.

5. Broil halibut fillets 8 minutes in the prepared oven, or until easily flaked with a fork.

6. Spread with the Parmesan cheese mixture, and continue broiling 2 minutes, or until topping is bubbly and lightly browned.

Toscana Soup

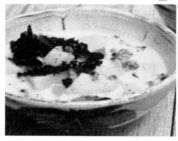

Prep Time: 10 mins **Cook Time:** 20 mins **Total Time:** 30 mins

MAKES 4 SERVINGS

INGREDIENTS

- ➢ 1 Lb. Ground Italian Sausage
- ➢ 4 Slices Thick-Cut Bacon, Diced
- ➢ 1 Small Onion, Diced
- ➢ 5 Cups Chicken Broth
- ➢ 2 Cups Water
- ➢ 5 Cups Cauliflower Florets, Medium-Sized Head Of Cauliflower
- ➢ 1 1/2 Cups Chopped Kale
- ➢ 1 Cup Heavy Cream Salt and Pepper To Taste
- ➢ Pinch Of Red Pepper Flakes
- ➢ Parmesan Cheese For Serving

INSTRUCTIONS

1. In a large dutch oven or stock, pot brown the sausage

until crumbled and cooked through.

2. Use a slotted spoon to remove the sausage to a paper towel-lined plate and set it aside.

3. Turn the pot to medium-high heat and add the bacon, cooking until fat is rendered and bacon begins to crisp. Add the onion and cook an additional 2 to 3 minutes.

4. Return the sausage to the pot and pour in the chicken broth, water, and cauliflower florets. Bring mixture to a boil, then reduce heat to simmer, cover, and cook for 10 minutes, until the cauliflower is fork-tender.

5. Stir in the kale and let cook an additional 2 minutes until softened slightly. Finally stir in the heavy cream, salt, and pepper to taste and the red pepper flakes.

6. Simmer for 2 more minutes until heated through. Enjoy with fresh parmesan on top.

Vietnamese Beef Noodles Soup

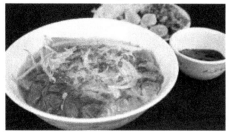

Prep Time: 15 mins **Cook Time:** 3hr **Total Time:** 3 hr 15 mins

MAKES 4 SERVINGS

INGREDIENTS

- ➢ 5-6 beef soup bones browned and roasted
- ➢ 1/2 Onion charred
- ➢ 1 tablespoon Fresh Ginger sliced
- ➢ 1 tbsp Salt
- ➢ 3 tbsp Fish Sauce
- ➢ 2 pods Star Anise
- ➢ 1 gallon Water

INSTRUCTIONS

1. Preheat oven to 425 degrees F.
2. Cover beef bones in water and boil for 15 minutes in a large stockpot on the stovetop while the oven preheats. Discard water.
3. Place parboiled beef bones and onion on a baking sheet

or casserole dish and roast for 45 -60 minutes, until bones are browned and onion is blackened.

4. Toss bones, onion, fresh ginger, salt, fish sauce, star anise, and freshwater into the pressure cooker. Set pressure cooker to high pressure for 2 hours. If you are using a stoveto

5. p, you will simmer for 6-8 hours instead.

6. Strain broth with a fine colander. Place shirataki noodles and meat of choice in a bowl, pour broth over the top into the bowl while it is still very hot.

7. Stir and let sit until raw meat is no longer pink and noodles are cooked 1 to 2 minutes.

8. Serve with condiments and veggies of choice on the side.

Sheet Pan Baked Tilapia with Roasted Vegetable

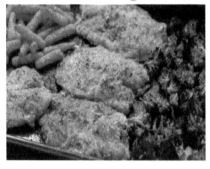

Prep Time: 10 mins **Cook Time:** 15 mins **Total Time:** 25 mins

MAKES 2 SERVINGS

INGREDIENTS

- ➤ 4 6 ounce tilapia fillets
- ➤ 3 cups broccoli florets, cut into 1-inch pieces
- ➤ 1 yellow squash, sliced
- ➤ 1 1/2 cups carrots, thinly sliced
- ➤ 4 Tablespoons olive oil
- ➤ 2 Tablespoons lemon juice
- ➤ 1 Tablespoon garlic, minced
- ➤ 1 Tablespoon fresh parsley
- ➤ 1/4 teaspoon dried red pepper flakes
- ➤ 1/4 teaspoon onion powder
- ➤ Salt & pepper

INSTRUCTIONS

1. Preheat oven to 400 degrees F.
2. Place veggies on a baking sheet and drizzle with 2 tablespoons olive oil. Sprinkle with salt and pepper, mix, and then push to the sides of the pan. In a small bowl, mix the remaining 2 tablespoons of olive oil, lemon juice, garlic, parsley, red pepper flakes, and onion powder.
3. Place tilapia on the pan between the veggies and rub the marinade on all sides of the fillets.
4. Sprinkle tilapia with salt and pepper.
5. Bake for 12-15 minutes or until fish reaches 145 degrees F and flakes easily.
6. Serve immediately.

Chicken Piccata

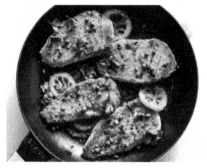

Prep Time: 30mins **Cook Time:** 20 min **Total Time**: 50 mins

MAKES 4 SERVINGS

INGREDIENTS

- ➢ 1 lemon
- ➢ 1 pound boneless skinless chicken breasts
- ➢ ¼ cup all-purpose flour
- ➢ ½ teaspoon salt
- ➢ ½ teaspoon ground pepper
- ➢ 1 tablespoon plus
- ➢ 4 teaspoons extra-virgin olive oil, divided
- ➢ 1 large sweet onion, sliced
- ➢ 1 clove garlic, minced
- ➢ 1 cup reduced-sodium chicken broth
- ➢ ¼ cup dry white wine
- ➢ 4 teaspoons drained capers
- ➢ ¼ cup chopped parsley

INSTRUCTIONS

Prepare Lemon and Chicken:

1. Cut lemon in half. Juice half of it, and cut the remaining half into thin slices.
2. Cut chicken breasts into 8 thin cutlets. Dredge Chicken: Whisk flour, salt, and pepper in a shallow dish or pie plate. Dredge chicken in the flour mixture, turning to coat.
3. Discard 2 teaspoons dredging flour and reserve the rest to thicken the sauce in step 5.

Brown Chicken:

1. Heat 2 teaspoons oil in a large non-stick skillet over medium-high heat. Add half the chicken and cook until the bottom is browned, 2 to 4 minutes. Turn over and continue cooking until browned on the bottom, 2 to 3 minutes. Set aside on a plate.
2. Repeat with 2 teaspoons oil and the remaining 4 pieces of dredged chicken, adjusting the heat to medium-low to prevent the chicken from burning.
3. Transfer the second batch of chicken to the plate.

Cook Onions and Garlic:

1. Wipe out the skillet with a clean paper towel. Add the

remaining 1 tablespoon oil and place the skillet over medium-high heat. Add onion, and cook, stirring often until soft and browned 5 to 7 minutes.

2. Add garlic, and cook, stirring constantly until the garlic is fragrant and just starting to brown, 30 to 90 seconds.

Make Sauce:

1. Sprinkle the remaining dredging flour over the onion mixture and stir to coat.
2. Stir in broth, white wine, capers, lemon slices, and lemon juice, increase heat to high and bring to a simmer, stirring constantly.

Finish Dish:

1. Add the chicken and any accumulated juices from the plate to the skillet and turn to coat in the sauce.
2. Bring to a simmer while turning the chicken in the sauce until the sauce is thickened, and the chicken is completely cooked through and hot, 3 to 4 minutes.
3. Stir in parsley, remove from the heat and serve.

Beef Tenderloin

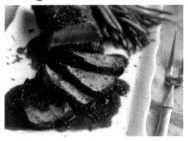

Prep Time: 15 mins **Cook Time:** 45 mins **Total Time:** 1 hr

MAKES 4 SERVINGS

INGREDIENTS

- ➢ 1 beef tenderloin Plan two 2″ filets per person
- ➢ 1 tablespoon Stone House Seasoning Recipe

INSTRUCTIONS

1. Place beef tenderloin on a rimmed baking sheet, pat dry with paper towels, and season both sides of the meat with Stone House Seasoning. Cover tightly with plastic wrap and refrigerate for one hour or up to 4 days before you plan on cooking and serving.

2. Remove from the refrigerator, unwrap and allow to stand for about an hour to come to room temperature.

3. Meanwhile, preheat grill or oven to approximately 400° F. Place tenderloin onto the grill or in the oven.

4. Allow the beef tenderloin to cook until it reaches 145° F

when checked with an internal meat thermometer in the thinner areas and 140° F in the thicker area, about 45 minutes.

5. Remove from grill and cover loosely with aluminum foil and allow to rest on the carving board for about 15 minutes before carving and serving.

Roasted Cauliflower

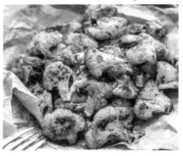

Prep Time: 15 mins **Cook Time:** 40 mins **Total Time:** 45 mins

MAKES 6 SERVINGS

INGREDIENTS

- 1 large head of cauliflower, cut into bite-sized florets (6-8 cups)
- 3 Tablespoons olive oil
- 1/4 teaspoon salt
- 1/4 teaspoon pepper
- 1 teaspoon oregano
- 1/4 teaspoon onion salt
- 1/4 teaspoon garlic powder
- 1/4 teaspoon dried basil

INSTRUCTIONS

1. Preheat the oven to 425 degrees.
2. Line a sheet pan with foil. Pour the oil over the

cauliflower florets in a large bowl.

3. Toss or stir to coat all the pieces. Mix all the seasonings. Sprinkle half the mixture on top of the cauliflower.

4. Toss and stir to coat. Sprinkle the remaining seasonings on top and stir again.

5. Place the cauliflower on the prepared sheet pan. Make sure the flat sides of the cauliflower are face down on the pan and that the cauliflower is now crowded. Bake for 15 minutes.

6. Remove the pan from the oven and use a spatula to flip the pieces of cauliflower over. Return the pan to the oven and bake for an additional 20 minutes.

7. Serve immediately.

Korean Beef

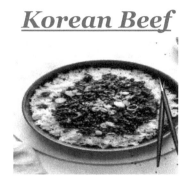

Prep Time: 10 mins **Cook Time:** 10 mins **Total Time:** 20 mins

MAKES 6 SERVINGS

INGREDIENTS

Sauce:

- ¼ cup reduced-sodium soy sauce (or use a gluten-free alternative and add salt as needed)
- 1 tablespoon honey or a liquid sugar-free alternative
- 1 teaspoon cornstarch ½ teaspoon crushed red pepper flakes

Stir-Fry:

- 2 tablespoons avocado oil
- 1 lb. lean ground beef (85/15)
- 1 tablespoon minced fresh garlic
- 1 tablespoon minced fresh ginger root

To Finish The Dish:

- ➢ 1 tablespoon sesame oil
- ➢ ¼ cup thinly sliced green onions, green parts only

INSTRUCTIONS

1. In a small bowl, prepare the sauce by whisking together the soy sauce, honey, cornstarch, and red pepper flakes. Set aside.
2. In a large skillet, heat the oil over medium-high heat.
3. Add the beef and cook, stirring, until no longer pink, breaking it up into crumbles as you cook, about 5 minutes.
4. Drain the beef. Return to the skillet. Add the garlic and the ginger to the skillet and cook, stirring, for 1 minute.
5. Stir the sauce into the beef.
6. Cook 2 more minutes, until heated through and the sauce thickens.
7. Off heat, drizzle the dish with sesame oil, sprinkle it with green onions, and serve.

French Toast

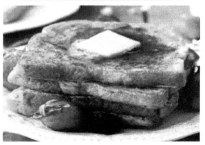

Prep Time: 5 mins **Cook Time:** 5 mins **Total Time:** 10 mins

MAKES 4 SERVINGS

INGREDIENTS

- ➤ 2 large eggs
- ➤ 1 cup milk, half and half, coconut milk, or almond milk
- ➤ Pinch salt
- ➤ 1 tablespoon granulated sugar, honey, or maple syrup
- ➤ 1 teaspoon vanilla extract
- ➤ 1 teaspoon ground cinnamon
- ➤ 8 slices sandwich bread Butter

INSTRUCTIONS

1. Whisk together eggs, milk, salt, sugar, vanilla, and cinnamon in a flat-bottomed pie plate or baking dish.
2. Place bread slices, one or two at a time, into the egg mixture and flip to make sure both sides of bread are well-coated.

3. Melt butter in a large skillet or on a griddle.
4. Place bread slices in skillet or on the griddle and cook on medium heat until golden brown on each side, about 2-3 minutes.
5. Serve immediately or keep warm in the oven until ready to serve, but no longer than about 30 minutes.

Sheet Pan Teriyaki Salmon

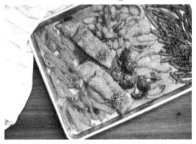

Prep Time: 10 mins **Cook Time:** 20 mins **Total Time:** 30 mins

MAKES 4 SERVINGS

INGREDIENTS

- ➢ 3 - 4 (6-ounce) salmon fillets
- ➢ 1 pound green beans ends trimmed
- ➢ 1 tablespoon olive oil
- ➢ 1/2 teaspoon kosher salt
- ➢ 1/2 teaspoon freshly ground black pepper
- ➢ 6 - 8 tablespoons teriyaki sauce + more if desired

INSTRUCTIONS

1. preheat oven to 425°F.
2. Line a rimmed baking sheet with parchment paper.
3. Arrange salmon fillets on the lined sheet pan and arrange green beans around the salmon.
4. Drizzle the olive oil over the green beans and sprinkle the green beans and salmon with salt and pepper.

5. Spread the teriyaki sauce, about 2 tablespoons per fillet, over the salmon. Bake the salmon and green beans until the salmon easily flakes with a fork, about 15 minutes.

6. Remove from the oven and drizzle with additional teriyaki sauce, if desired.

Lemon Basil Chicken

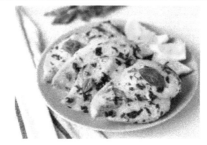

Prep Time: 15 mins **Cook Time:** 15 **Total Time:** 30 mins

MAKES 4 SERVINGS

INGREDIENTS

- ➢ 1 tablespoon extra-virgin olive oil
- ➢ 1/2 large yellow onion finely chopped, about
- ➢ 1 cup 4 cloves garlic minced
- ➢ 1 1/2 pounds boneless skinless chicken breasts, cut into
- ➢ 3/4-inch pieces
- ➢ 2 tablespoons low-sodium soy sauce
- ➢ 1/4 teaspoon ground black pepper
- ➢ 5 cups loosely packed baby spinach about
- ➢ 5 ounces 1 tablespoon lemon zest
- ➢ 2 tablespoons lemon juice
- ➢ 2 cups fresh basil leaves
- ➢ Kosher salt and pepper to taste
- ➢ Prepared brown rice for serving

INSTRUCTIONS

1. In a large skillet, heat the olive oil over medium.

2. Once hot, add the onion and cook, stirring often until softened, about 4 minutes.

3. Add the garlic and cook until fragrant, about 30 additional seconds.

4. Add the chicken, increase the heat to medium-high, and let cook for 3 minutes, browning all sides.

5. Stir in the soy sauce and black pepper. Let cook until the chicken is completely cooked through, about 3 minutes longer.

6. Stir in the spinach a few handfuls at a time, letting the heat of the pan wilt it as you go. Stir in the lemon zest, lemon juice, and basil.

7. Cook and stir just until the basil is wilted about 1 additional minute.

8. Taste and season with additional salt or pepper as desired. Serve warm with rice as desired.